Navigating the Fog of Dementia

The Agony of Being a Caregiver

By

Sandra Olson

This book is copywritten in June 2025
All rights are held by Sandra Olson
Copying requires written permission from the author.

Table of Contents

Prologue ---When Memory Fades

Chapter 1 --- Understanding the Fog – Dementia Demystified

Chapter2 --- The Daily Dance – Practical Care Strategies

Chapter 3 --- Emotional Rollercoaster – Supporting Your Loved One

Chapter 4 --- Caring for Yourself

Chapter 5 --- Some Personal Insights

Prologue---When Memory Fades

The day my mother turned against me was the day everything changed. It wasn't dramatic –no sudden collapse or tearful revelation. Suddenly she was no longer my loving, sweet mother but a vengeful stranger. In my sixty-eight years as her daughter nor in the seventeen years she had lived with me had I seen this person. She shouted and glared at me with accusing eyes. She was adamant that the grandchild who had visited us had stolen her hairbrush and left a fake in its place. She shook the offending hairbrush in my face. There was no reasoning with her. This was the first of many hurtful episodes. After a nap, she remembered nothing of the episode. To her it was a blackout. To keep from blaming her or being angry, we named this other 'person' her 'evil twin'. But the hurt was hard to ignore.

And so began our journey into the fog of dementia – a path that would challenge everything I thought I knew about love, patience and the unbreakable bonds of family. This book is for you – the sons, daughters, spouses, and friends who find themselves thrust into the role of caregiver. It's a roadmap for the rocky terrain ahead, filled with practical advice I wish I had from the start. But more than that, it's a reminder that you're not alone on this journey.

We had all know for months that my mother was losing her memory. When she was diagnosed with vascular dementia it didn't come as a complete shock. I'm a nurse and the signs were obvious. But I mainly worked in Obstetrics and was not prepared for the road ahead. Even geriatric nurses are given little practical knowledge for something so intimate as a family member going through this fog. I did some things wrong, but also discovered some things that worked for us.

I don't know if it holds true in all cases, but her family doctor told us that the main difference he had noted between Alzheimer's and dementia was that those with Alzheimer's didn't know they were losing their memory, while dementia patients knew the horror of losing themselves.

So, I will try to shed some light on this disease for you that I have discovered on this journey. It will not be an easy path, but it can be accomplished with dignity for all involved.

Your experiences will not exactly mirror mine, but mine may help you understand some of what is happening to your loved one.

Chapter 1 –Understanding the Fog –Dementia Demystified

When Mom was first diagnosed, I felt overwhelmed by medical jargon even thou I am a nurse. Take a deep breath. You don't need to become a neurologist overnight. Focus on understanding how the symptoms affect your loved one's daily behavior and the care they need.

Here are a few facts for background information. Currently more than 55 million people have dementia worldwide. Every year, there are nearly 10 million new cases. Dementia results from a variety of diseases and injuries that affect the brain. This damage interferes with the ability of brain cells to communicate with each other. When brain cells cannot communicate normally, thinking, behavior and feelings can be affected.

Dementia affects a person's executive functioning, making it challenging for them to complete simple tasks, and the steps that go into them, such as having a shower or getting dressed.

One of the most common signs of early-stage Alzheimer's disease and dementia is forgetting recently learned information, including forgetting important dates or events, asking the same questions over and over, and increasingly needing to rely on memory aids or family members for things they used to handle on their own. With normal ageing we may forget something but will remember it later. Dementia makes it almost impossible to remember the information they are seeking.

Agitation that may happen with dementia due to can seem like it comes out of nowhere, and each person's experience can be drastically different. The condition can be broken down into three distinct categories, each with their own set of behaviour challenges.

Restlessness includes pacing or rocking, jumpiness, irritability, wandering or hoarding.

Verbal aggression includes screaming, swearing, complaining, being negative, emotional outbursts, repetitive questions and sentences.

Physical aggression can include hitting, biting, kicking, throwing things, resisting help or hurting themselves.

Those with dementia may experience changes in their ability to develop and follow a plan or work with numbers. They may have trouble following a familiar recipe or keeping track of monthly bills. They may have difficulty concentrating and take much longer to do things than they did before. While occasional problems with finances is normal, they often make poor financial decisions and become easy targets for scams. They may lose things and be unable to go back over their steps to find the lost item and will accuse others of stealing, especially as the disease progresses.

During her 'spells' my mother fixated on her bank account and was certain money was missing. She hid her checkbook and purse, believing that someone was stealing from her account, and usually that person was me.

Early dementia causes difficulty with driving to even familiar locations, with remembering rules of a game or how to use the normally familiar electronic devices. People with dementia often experience changes in their emotional responses and may have less control over their feelings and how to express them. They may overreact to things, have rapid mood changes, feel irritable, or become distant or uninterested in things.

For nine years mother lived in a house attached to ours. We had a door between our living rooms so I could care for her everyday as needed and she ate dinner with us each night. When she became increasingly forgetful, we worried she would leave a stove burner on until a fire started, and we began making plans to build a new home where she would live with us. As we began downsizing for the move she started having crying spells. Getting rid of extra furniture that she would no longer need was especially hard. She would have a huge bedroom with a sitting room in the new house and a private bathroom, but she had a hard time grasping how it would work.

In the earlier stages, memory loss and confusion may be mild. The person may be aware of — and frustrated by — the changes happening to them. They have difficulty recalling recent events, making decisions or processing what was said by others. In the later stages, memory loss becomes far more severe to the point where even loved family members can become strangers to them. They may forget names and faces.

We were lucky in this respect because Mom never forgot her people. She recognized family members including grandchildren and would ask me how they were doing. True, she would ask repeatedly then couldn't remember my answer, but she remembered them by name.

Friends have told me how depressing it was for them when their parent or spouse didn't remember who they were. I didn't have to face that problem.

A person with late-stage dementia may show distress by crying, pacing, screaming or shouting. This may be due to fear, anxiety, depression or difficulty understanding what is happening.

When my mother had crying spells, she didn't know why she was crying. If I asked her what was wrong or what I could do to help, she would shrug and cry harder. All I could do was hug and comfort her until the spell was over.

Dementia causes loss of the ability to keep track of dates, seasons and the passage of time. They may forget where they are or how they got there.

At times Mom would wake up frightened and she didn't know where she was. Pointing out familiar objects and furniture in her room often helped her recognize her place. It was easier for her to remember her childhood home than it was to recognize her own bedroom.

Dementia causes trouble following or joining a conversation, often make the person stop in middle of a sentence and have no idea how to continue. They repeat themselves and ask the same questions over and over as short-term memory becomes almost non-existent.

They struggle with vocabulary and have trouble naming familiar objects or will use the wrong name. As a result, they may withdraw from hobbies, social activities or other engagements. They may have trouble keeping up with a favorite sports team or watching a favorite television show.

All this sounds frightening, and people often wonder if dementia is hereditary. As far as science can determine, the majority of dementia is not inherited by children or grandchildren. In rarer types of dementia there may be a strong genetic link, but these are only a tiny proportion of overall cases of dementia.

Chapter 2 – The Daily Dance --- Practical Care Strategies

Caring for someone with dementia requires a delicate balance of assistance and allowing some independence. Here are a few strategies I've found helpful:

Create a Dementia-Friendly Environment

- Reduce clutter: A tidy space helps reduce confusion
- Improve lighting: Good lighting can prevent falls and reduce agitation
- Use labels: Clear, large-print labels on drawers and cabinets can help maintain some independence

Establish Routines

Consistency is key. Try to:
- Keep mealtimes, bedtimes, and bathing schedules consistent
- Break tasks into simple steps
- Allow extra time for activities and encourage participation
- Soft music can be calming
- Provide a time for rest and a nap

Communication Tips

- Speak clearly and slowly

- Use simple words and short sentences
- Be patient and offer reassurance
- Avoid arguing or correcting mistakes

Watch for infections which can make confusion worse. I'm not sure why it happens but when the body is stressed because of a urinary tract infection, a cold, yeast infection, or diarrhea, the brain becomes even more confused. Encourage fluid intake to prevent dehydration which also stresses the brain. Make certain normal medications are taken on time; missing blood pressure or heart medications, meds for diabetes or a chronic medical condition stresses the brain as well as the body.

Try to determine what helps your person relax. My mother was raised on a farm, and I found frequent drives through the countryside helped tremendously. She would return home ready to nap or at least rest. During one long crying jag, we went to McDonalds and ate French fries in the car and that cured the spell.

Some treatment options can consist of cognition enhancing medications but take care to watch for side effects.

No cure exists, but medications and management strategies may temporarily improve symptoms.

Cognition-enhancing medication can improve mental function, lower blood pressure, and may balance mood.

Memantine is used to slow the neurotoxicity involved in Alzheimer disease, dementia and other neurodegenerative diseases. Memantine is in a class of medications called NMDA receptor antagonists. It works by decreasing abnormal activity in the brain.

Memantine is not a cure for dementia, but it can help with symptoms like being forgetful, feeling confused or feeling anxious. The most common side effects of memantine are feeling sleepy or dizzy, headaches, constipation and shortness of breath.

Rivastigmine is used to treat mild to moderate dementia associated with Alzheimer's disease or Parkinson's disease. Rivastigmine will not cure or stop the disease from getting worse, however, rivastigmine can improve the thinking ability in some patients. Rivastigmine may cause nausea, vomiting, diarrhea, stomach pain, loss of appetite, or weight loss, trouble urinating.

Donepezil or Aricept is a medication that works by improving attention, memory and the ability to engage in daily activities. Side effects include diarrhea, nausea, headache, dizziness, fatigue, indigestion, muscle cramps, seizures.

Rexulti is one of the newer drugs and was not available when we needed it. Side effects can be severe and include stroke, tardive dyskinesia and hyperglycemia.

The doctor never put my mother on any of these meds because her advanced age made it more likely that she would have severe side-effects. She was on a dose of Prozac which seemed to help some. Each person is different, and the pros and cons need to be tailored for them.

Chapter 3 – Emotional Rollercoaster – Supporting Your Loved One

Remember people with dementia will experience some or all of these symptoms:

Cognitive: mental decline and memory loss, confusion especially in the evening hours, (called 'sundowner's symptoms'), disorientation, inability to speak or understand language, making things up, or inability to recognize common things. Looping is very common in dementia. It can involve the repeating of stories or fixations. How you approach it and/or embrace it makes a world of difference in your interaction with the individual. Allow it to happen and you can have a deeper, richer interaction with your loved one.

Behavioral: irritability, personality changes, restlessness, lack of restraint, or wandering and getting lost. Many people with dementia become restless and may fidget or pace up and down. They may constantly wring their hands, pull at their clothes or touch themselves inappropriately in public. This could be because of pain or discomfort, needing the toilet, a need for more physical activity or problems with their environment.

Mother's personality changes were the most shocking for me. She would yell or become angry for no reason. Sometimes she would wake up and not recognize where she was, and it would frighten her into a crying spell. Other times she was certain that people were making fun of her, and her feelings were hurt.

Mood: anxiety, loneliness, mood swings, or nervousness. For many caregivers, there comes a time when the loved one almost seems to be their shadow. As the caregiver moves around the house or apartment, the loved one stays right alongside as if they are afraid to be alone. It can be challenging to the caregiver to have any personal space.

Mother was normally friendly and out-going, but now she often became withdrawn and anxious around other people and only wanted to be with me or my husband. Other times she didn't want anyone at all to be near her.

Psychological: depression, hallucination, or paranoia.

The first hallucinations my mother experienced were auditory. She would ask why no one was answering the phone when it wasn't ringing. Later she would see people who weren't there. She became positive people were stealing from her. It was especially hard when her paranoia focused on me. She would approach my husband and tell him not to let me go to her bank.

Muscular: inability to combine muscle movements or unsteady walking or falling.

Mother became clumsy and fell often. She needed a walker but would sometimes park it and try to walk by grabbing on to furniture or walls. She constantly had multiple head bruises. One time she laughed and said she hit her head so often because she was "top heavy".

Also common: jumbled speech, or sleep disorder, confusion about dates and times. Try to avoid delving into past unpleasant memories. Don't remind your loved one that someone they knew and cared for has passed away. Avoid quizzing them on past experiences but allow them to talk about pleasant things from their past, even repeatedly.

Every time we went for a drive in the country, my mother told me how her father took them for drives every Sunday. She would expound on what a great father he was, and I just smiled and nodded. She talked about the fun things she did as a child on the farm, and it made her so happy to remember the past that I didn't have the heart to stop the repeated conversations.

Non-drug approaches to managing behavior symptoms promote physical and emotional comfort.
Steps to developing successful non-drug treatments include:

- Recognize that the person is not just "acting mean or ornery," but is having further symptoms of the disease. It's their "evil twin".
- Identify the cause of the confusion as it relates to the experiences of the person with dementia. They may

not recognize that they are hungry or need to use the restroom.

- Change the environment only to resolve challenges and obstacles to comfort, security and ease of mind. Keep things as normal as possible without making big changes to their living space. Make sure there are non-slip rugs or no rugs at all if they are a fall risk. Let them have their favorite keepsakes and familiar furnishings.

Coping tips

Monitor personal comfort. Often the person cannot describe what is bothering them. Check for pain, hunger, thirst, constipation, full bladder, fatigue, infections and skin irritation. Maintain a comfortable room temperature.

Avoid being confrontational or arguing about facts. For example, if a person expresses a wish to go visit a parent who died years ago, don't point out that the parent is dead. Express that a visit would be nice at a future date but is not feasible at this time.

I was not aware of this and would often remind Mom that her parents were no longer alive when she asked to go live with them. Luckily this didn't seem to bother her, and she would accept the truth for a while.

Redirect the person's attention. Try to remain flexible, patient and supportive by responding to the emotion, not the behavior. Offering a snack, a television program, or going for a walk or drive can help redirect them.

Create a calm environment. Avoid noise, glare, insecure space and too much background distraction, including television. Sometimes returning to a quieter space is the best solution.

My mother often preferred the quiet of her room if company visited our house.

Allow adequate rest between stimulating events. Encourage naps often.

Provide a security object. Did the person have a pet that is not available now? There are special 'toy' dogs and cats on the market that provide comfort for the elderly.

My mother's friend had a toy dog that moved, barked and snuggled. They both thought it was alive and never wondered why it didn't need to eat or go outside..

Acknowledge requests and respond to them. All of us know how frustrating it is to wait for something.

Look for reasons behind each behavior. Is the person frustrated by something currently happening? Be sure to consult a physician to identify any causes related to medication side effects or illness.

Explore various solutions until you stumble on one that works! Be creative. If the stress becomes too much, maybe a care facility is the answer. 60% of caregivers ruin their own health by struggling to care for a loved one too long. Try not to feel guilty if this becomes the best option for you.

As my mother's angry spells became more frequent, I found myself having bouts of depression and PTSD. When she began demanding that she have her own apartment, we used this as the time to move her into an assisted living facility. She made friends there and received excellent care. Within twelve months, her symptoms increased so much that she had to be moved into their locked down memory care unit.

Don't take the behavior personally. This is especially hard and sometimes sharing your experiences with others can help you cope.

You'll find as I did that many others have gone through this trial, and they can be a great support for you. I sometimes needed to visit a friend where I could cry on her understanding shoulders.

Chapter 4 ---Caring for Yourself

Don't try to do everything by yourself. Enlist help from other family members or friends. Caregiving is a stressful situation both mentally and physically. You'll find that the time will come when you can't leave a dementia person alone. Don't expect to provide twenty-four-hour care by yourself. You'll end up making yourself sick!

My husband and I struggled to take care of my mother. Even when she was mostly lucid and seemed fairly normal, we found that if left alone she would do things like climb on a stool to reach something on a high shelf. Or decide to drive herself to the store. We ended up selling her car and turning in her driver's license for a state ID card. It was hard to limit her activities, but it was the only way to keep her safe.

Mom could make herself breakfast of cereal and yogurt, but I made her lunch, and she came to my house for dinner. As we discovered her still trying to cook, we moved her in with us to prevent a fire or accident.

Check in your area for caregiver support groups. Most towns have them. They can be a wonderful source of information and support. Just knowing that you are not the only one experiencing this painful situation can help.

Caregiver support groups are a way for you and other caregivers to share experiences, insight, and words of encouragement. Whether you're an in-home caregiver caring for someone with Alzheimer's or another form of dementia, or have a family member in an assisted living community, a caregiver support group can help you cope and find solutions.

Check with your **Area Agency on Aging** for local groups.

Here are several online support groups:

Memory People ---
www.facebook.com/groups/180666768616259

Dementia Caregivers Support Group-
www.facebook.com/groups/672984902717938

Caring for a Spouse with Dementia --
www.facebook.com/groups/275900859414999

Caring for Elderly Parents—
www.facebook.com/groups/113354218750970

Chapter 5---Some Personal Insights

I'm including some excerpts from my diary just to show how things happened for us with my mother's dementia. Her memory loss had been going on for several years before this, but these notes show the downward spiral. (I've removed the names of family members and friends for their privacy.)

---

15 April 2019

We've finally figured out more about Mom's 'angry spells' as she calls them. She probably has Dementia Psychosis.

She gets angry, paranoid, and mean when they happen. She yells, cries and sometimes starts shaking all over.

She looks at you with hate in her eyes and pushes you away. She'll go into her bedroom and shut the door and brood. If we leave her alone or she takes a nap, she eventually comes out of it. The next day she doesn't remember anything…there is a blank spot in her memory. A blackout.

She's done this off and on since the stress of moving last summer. Mostly they are directed at me, but last month she yelled at Ron for nothing, and he finally knows how it feels. They seem to happen every few weeks now. It makes it a little easier to cope with now that we know what the spells are, but it's still hard not to get your feelings hurt when she is yelling at you for something you didn't do.

She went in her room and wouldn't come out for lunch. I ended up going to my friend K's house to cry on her shoulder. Her mother had spells like this before she died. Boy is it hard to deal with!! They seem to be coming more often now.

I forgot to mention that we finally found the missing Christmas presents that she hid. The gloves and lotion were in the bottom drawer of her dresser under clothes she doesn't wear right now. I found the blouses on the bottom shelf in the back of her television console. Go figure!

19 April 2019

Mom had a horrible day today. She accused me of trying to steal all her money and she asked Ron to not let me go to the bank to take it. She yelled at me, and I had to leave the house to cry.

While Ron and I ran an errand she called S and told her I was trying to take her money, and she wanted S to come from Texas to get her.

This is so horrible I can't stand it! She probably won't remember any of it tomorrow, but I feel like she's stabbed me in the heart. My blood pressure was 194/121 and I had to take extra medicine to lower it.

This is the second one this week, so they are coming more often now.

12 May 2029 ---Mother's Day

Mom ended up collapsing the night of her spell and we had to call the ambulance to take her to the hospital.

Her blood pressure was so low they kept her overnight to hydrate her with IV fluids. She had the spell because she didn't eat or drink anything and got dehydrated. I actually found her lunch in the trash. She acted like she thought the food might be poisoned.

We went to see Dr. P the following Monday and he prescribed a low dose of Prozac. It's been almost a month, and she hasn't had another spell. (We started calling it her 'evil twin' so we could separate the real Mom from the crazy one.)

---

8 July 2019

Mom had been doing better for a while, but now her dementia is worse. On Friday when I came back from my early morning walk at 6:30 she was lying on the floor in the dining room crying and shaking all over. She hadn't used her cane or walker and was totally confused. She kept saying "Don't leave me alone."

(Needless to say, I don't dare go walking in the morning anymore. She used to stay in bed until at least 7A and by then I was back.) I got her settled back in bed and she said she didn't think she fell, just laid down on the floor. Wrong. For two days after that she complained that the hip, she had surgery on, hurt and so did her wrist. So, I'm sure she fell. We put a heat pack on it, and she took Tylenol. I didn't see any bruising, but it could have been deep. Yesterday her hip was better, so I think she just bruised it, and we didn't go to the doctor.

Last night she got up at midnight to 'hunt' for two pairs of brown slacks. (They are way too big, and she had given them to me to give to Goodwill, so I'd put them in my closet.) Ron told her I was sleeping and to go back to bed, which she did until 2 o'clock. Then she got up and wandered around until he made her go back to bed and he went to bed. Evidently, she got back up sometime later because she left a flashlight out in the dining room. She told me this morning, she got up to sleep on the brown couch because she couldn't fall asleep in her bed, and she used the flashlight to see the clock.

Since we were both asleep, I'm just glad she didn't decide to go outdoors or fall again. This morning, she was up at 6:30 w/o a cane or walker. She told me she wanted the brown slacks, so I gave them back to her and she hung them up in the closet.

She ate breakfast then was upset that her newspaper wasn't here yet.
After breakfast I talked her into getting a bath but now, she was upset because she couldn't find the yellow slacks she was sure should be in her closet!! (When she gets upset like this, she is certain I have hidden whatever it is she is looking for.) She has never had a pair of yellow pants that I know of. I convinced her that the new pair of white & beige striped pants was the one she was looking for and she finally accepted that.

When she doesn't get enough sleep, she is very hard to deal with, so I guess now she needs a sleeping pill every night.

12 August 2019

We had Mom's 90th Birthday party last Monday.

S came from Texas and K came from Ohio to be here. It was a little crowded, but I slept on the couch bed and gave K my room. It worked out fine. We had the party at the Stone Meadow Clubhouse with K's family, G, K, and A came up from Conway with her friend E. Even B and R T came. We had a lovely time and Mom was pleased. She did have one of her spells on the last day K was here, but after ten days of being off her schedule, it was expected. (She thought Ron and K were making fun of her and it made her cry. Of course, they weren't at all. Sigh.)

Today when we came home from church Mom was upset again. She said she's going to visit S next time K wants to come to visit because she doesn't want to see her. She gets upset with me when I try to convince her Ron & K weren't making fun of her. It doesn't make any sense and she's very spiteful about her accusations.

I don't know how long this visit from the 'evil twin' will last. But poor Ron feels hurt.

27 September 2019

Mom is getting weaker and weaker.

She is having more trouble getting a bath; even with her electric bath chair I have to help her in and out of the tub because her legs are so weak. She is having more of her 'blackout' spells and even the sleeping pills don't help much at night anymore. She wanders around at all hours of the night which is disruptive for us. Some mornings she gets up crying and shaking all over saying she wishes she could die because she is so tired of living. After I get her to eat a little and rest up, she feels better but complains about being tired all the time. She is losing interest in most things now and often just sits and thinks about her past (the way Daddy did). Other times she has a better day, and I take her riding in the car, or we all go out to lunch.

She is going to try a week at a nursing home for 'respite' care when Ron and I go for a little break at Branson. We've scouted out every place around here and of course they are all super expensive. $215/night.

She's talking about moving to a nursing home, but we want to find one that can watch over her well and that she will like. The place where she will go for the one week is lovely and seems to be willing to work with us.

(All of the places that do 'memory/dementia' care charge $6300/mon. I'm working with the VA to give her extra money to help cover the cost, but basically it will start using some of her savings.)

---

6 October 2019

Mom's been fussing about going for respite care now. She keeps saying she wants to die, and several times has asked me if I could get her some pills to take so she could die. I keep telling her they don't always work the way you want, and she could end up worse off that she is now; that I could go to jail for giving them to her and that we love her and that she will die when Heavenly Father chooses to take her.

She changes her mind about going to a nursing home constantly.

One day saying I should put her there because she doesn't know what she is doing and says mean things to us, other days she begs me not to leave her there.

When I took her on a tour of Village on the Park she got upset and said if she went there for a week that I wouldn't come back to get her. She is kind of driving me crazy with all this!

---

27 November 2019

Thanksgiving is tomorrow and there will be thirteen of us for dinner. Mom is already getting 'antsy' about having that many extra people in the house. She said she was going to lock her bedroom door so no one could steal anything. I get sooooo frustrated with her sometimes. I already have a ton of things to do without her freaking out on me.

Today she brought out an old blue plastic hairbrush — and insisted this was the brush A left when she 'stole' the good one from her. I kept trying to remain calm and explain it was probably a mistake, but she was getting more vocal about it until I snapped at her. I told her under no circumstance was she to mention this to A or I would put her in a nursing home! I took the brush and threw it in the trash. She wanted to confront A about something that she thinks happened five years ago!!

Mom has several hairbrushes that she uses every day. She could buy anything she wanted but gets upset over stupid things that she fixates on.

Of course, she got her feelings hurt and closed herself in her bedroom.

We had been having a good week before this. She hadn't gotten up one time during the night but said she wished she had died in her sleep. That has become a constant refrain for several months. But having company seems to push her over the edge.

30 November 2019

Mom did OK on Thursday because I gave her an extra dose of her Prozac. But Friday even after I bought her a brand-new hairbrush, she went off again when I was away from home. I took my granddaughter to the movies and when I came back, Ron said she was ranting about someone sneaking into her room on Thursday and stealing another hairbrush. Even he is losing patience with her.

When I confronted her and asked what hairbrush was missing, she went off on me. She started screaming and crying that she wanted to move out because I didn't believe her. She wanted boxes to pack up her stuff so to placate her I gave her two empty boxes and told her she could pack them. She slammed her door at me.

When W and C arrived, she begged them to take her back to Texas with them to S's house to live. Then she spent an hour crying and saying that I was kicking her out. I'd been messaging S about all of this, and she said she doesn't have a place for Mom to stay with her. So, I'm starting to look for a nursing home with a memory care unit. The problem so far is that they are supper expensive, between $6 and 7 thousand a month! That will take all her monthly income plus her savings. But I don't know what else to do.

4 December 2019

Saturday Mom was better and seemed cheerful. She went with us to the Bentonville Town Square to see the Christmas sales booths with W and C.

She was able to slowly walk around the whole square. Sunday when she woke up, she didn't remember Friday or most of Saturday at all. She asked if W and C had come to visit, and I told her about their visit and going to the square. She vaguely remembered some things but didn't remember Friday at all. When she asked about Friday, I told her she had a spell. She said, "Don't tell me what I did." I feel so bad for her. She is not responsible for the 'evil twin' and yet she drives everyone crazy when she has a spell.

W helped me get the Christmas tree down from the attic before they left for Siloam and Mom loved all the lights. They wanted to visit K before they left for home on Sunday morning.

Sunday afternoon I found Mom crying and she said she missed her family. All I could do was hug her and tell her I was sorry. How much worse is it going to be when she's not with me and Ron? She's lived with us for almost 20 years now.

I've been checking into more nursing homes. Some said she could stay in an assisted living area since she can take care of eating, bathing and getting around so well. They would move her to a memory care unit when she gets worse. She hated the respite memory unit because everyone was so much worse off that they couldn't even carry on a conversation with her. Some had to be fed and dressed. We'll see how that goes. I hate to put her anywhere and feel so guilty about it, but we can't go on this way. We never know when the spells will occur, we can't figure out if there is anything that triggers them…they just happen randomly. They are so hurtful and disruptive to us.

Having company seems to be a big stressor for her. Just thinking about the people coming for Thanksgiving had her nervous. She's already worried about Christmas and keeps asking who is coming.

We are also getting very nervous about leaving her alone when we go to church. One Sunday she had chest pain and told me she had to take a nitro pill before they went away. So, it is getting to the point where we have to do something as she can't be left alone.

We thought about trying to get someone to stay with her when we are away but worry that she could have a spell and frighten them. The nursing homes assure me that they know how to handle such things.

---

12 December 2019

This has been the hardest thing I've had to do in my life…harder than dealing with my miscarriage, my divorce and finding out K was going to prison. Putting Mom in an assisted living facility is worse because I feel so guilty. I always thought I would be able to take care of her and if I needed physical help, I could hire someone to come in and help with her, like we did with Daddy. I didn't count on her mind going before her body. It's hard living with someone who complains every day about being alive.

She will be moved in January to The Village on the Park Bentonville. It is less than two miles from our house and a wonderful facility. BUT she doesn't want to leave Ron and me. She has never lived alone and has been with us almost 20 years now.

Today I picked out a nice 1-bedroom apt. and put down the $1500 fee. It will cost around $4000 /month, but they provide all meals, laundry service, house cleaning, telephone and cable and medication administration. She has a view of the inside courtyard from her bedroom. There are tons of activities including a library, movie theater and bingo. Right now, she is bored at home with hardly any activities except TV with us in the evening and an occasional lunch at a restaurant.

I'm hoping this will give her more social stimulation, so she won't constantly be saying she wants to die. Every morning, she complains about still being alive. She asked Ron if he thought any of the tree branches out back would be strong enough for her to hang herself!

She will be allowed to leave the facility to go to lunch with us or spend a day here at the house.

We are allowed to come and have lunch with her at the facility.

Her room is close to the cafeteria and the nurse's station. They assured me they will encourage her to participate in activities like they did when she stayed for respite care. She didn't like being on that hall because no one could talk to her. They are too far into dementia or Alzheimer's over there, so she will be in an assisted living hall with lots of other folks who are more 'with it' and active.

We plan to go to the facilities "Winter Wonderland" luncheon on the 21st and Ron will be their Santa Claus for the activity. Hopefully she will meet a few people then and feel more comfortable about the move.

---

11 January 2020

Mom has finally accepted that she needs to move to the assisted living facility. She hasn't had a bad spell for a week and says she'll be fine if she can take all her things with her.

I made arrangements to have most of her bedroom furniture moved and her lift chair from our living room.

She will even be able to take her small organ. She was playing it again this week for the first time in weeks. Playing seems to calm her down.

One of the women we met at the lunch when Ron was Santa just moved there and she will help Mom settle in. She is very with-it and is one of their welcoming committee members. Her name is Polly. She was the only resident brave enough to sit on Santa's lap for a photo.

Mom's room is right across the hallway from their library and the main dining room is at the end of her hall, so she won't have to walk very far.

I'm still worried because lately she has been having more dizzy spells in the mornings. A few days ago, I caught her getting ready to climb on the stepstool to see what was on the top shelf of her closet!

The next day she fell and there is a huge bruise on her hip. She already had a sore spot on her ribs but doesn't remember how that happened.

If she falls over there, they will most likely make her go to the hospital for an x-ray. I hope that doesn't happen. I've been trying to get her to use her walker more often instead of just the cane, but she is resistant to the idea.

12 January 2020

This has been a horrible way to start my Sabbath morning. Mom is having one of her 'spells'. S is coming tonight to help pack her things this week and now it has become more real to her that she is going to move.

She's been ranting about how I "stole her $50,000 down payment on the house." "How I'm trying to get rid of her so A could live in her room!" (A has her own apartment.) None of it makes any sense because I also put down $50,000 and hers is at the mortgage company just like mine, and not in my bank account as she keeps saying. She refused to eat her breakfast and ended up throwing it in the trash when I wasn't in the kitchen.

If she doesn't eat and drink again, it will be like last time when she got dehydrated, fell and passed out, then ended up in the hospital getting fluids. I'm so upset I've been shaking. It's hard to watch her like this and even harder to be the one being verbally attacked all the time.

She snuck out to the hot tub and told Ron how much she "loved him", and that I'm a horrible daughter.

Now she's in her room bawling her eyes out that she must go away. She is going to the nicest, most expensive assisted living facility in the area but I'm still being mean to her. It is so hard to not get mad at her, but I know it's the spells…this "evil twin" is hard to deal with!

---

31 January 2020

S helped get Mom moved to the Village on the Park. She was impressed with the facility, too. Mom's apartment looks nice with her own furniture in it.

She has a private room with her own bathroom and a small kitchenette. She plays her organ every day, which is more than when she was here.

She walks in the halls for exercise. She has nutritious meals and if she doesn't like the scheduled meal she can order from a little menu. They clean her room and do her laundry and even change the bedding. The nurse gives her the medications.

She is making a few friends and has gone to their theater and played bingo.

Everyone who works there is friendly and helpful. She has had a few breakdowns with crying and wanting to come 'back home'. I visit her at least once every day. She can phone us whenever she wants and called three times one evening.

Yesterday I took her to Dr. M for a cortisone injection in her knee. It had been four months since the last one and it was hurting and 'giving out' on her at times. Before the appointment I brought her to the house to see Ron and we showed her that we have turned her old bedroom into a workroom. I have my sewing machine in there and Ron has a big table with computers. I'm hoping that will emphasize that her move is permanent. Hopefully she'll settle in soon.

---

15 February 2020

We've finally reached a milestone with Mom today.

At least I hope it's permanent. She came here for homemade soup for lunch and a visit.

One of her toes was hurting but otherwise she was upbeat. She enjoyed lunch and watching the birds at the feeder. When it came time to leave, we took a little drive first. She told me that she didn't feel like the house was her home anymore and it wasn't hard to leave it now. Her apartment is home. Thank goodness.

She still has her crying spells, and it worried the workers at the facility at first. But they see that it is temporary and not a sign of depression, just a symptom of the dementia. Mom will be sobbing one minute and fine the next. She enjoyed the Valentine Party they had yesterday even though I didn't attend with her. And she won a little prize at bingo.

On Thursday I went and had dinner with Mom for a special Italian Party they were having. And last week K and J had lunch with her. I think it makes her feel more like we are visiting her home for us to go there than to always bring her back here.

---

12 March 2020

Mom has settled in better at the Village, but her dementia is getting much worse.

She has crying jags most mornings now. Yesterday she called and wanted me to take her back to the doctor to 'fix' her. We had just seen Dr. P on Monday and I told her there was nothing that could make the dementia go away. She got mad and hung up on me. P has increased her Prozac now so maybe it will start to help a little. She is even more forgetful and can't remember what you tell her for ten minutes. She calls repeatedly to ask about appointments and when I'm coming over. I have to go over there at least once a day and sometimes more.

Two days ago, she seems to have started having the hallucinations again. She is positive an older "grandmotherly" woman came into her room at night to put her hands on her head and pray for her. She said it made her feel better. No one like that works there at night. I told her maybe it was her 'guardian angel'.

Today she has the beginnings of a chest cold. I got permission from the nurse to take her cold medicine, cough drops and soup. She plans to stay in her room so as not to make anyone else sick.

Right now, the whole nation is going crazy worried about this **coronavirus**. Tens of thousands of people have died in China, and it has spread to Europe and now the United States. We have six confirmed cases in AR, but there are hundreds of cases in New York, California, and Washington. It is basically a horrid chest infection, but it can kill people with compromised immune systems, heart disease, diabetes, lung disease and the elderly. It starts with a low-grade fever and the Village is screening everyone before they are allowed to visit.

12 April 2020 EASTER

We are all still stuck at home with no Church services. Listening to choral music and reading scriptures on our own. I have been reading from "Jesus the Christ" this week. It has a wonderful, detailed account of this Easter week.

I was allowed to see Mom today for the first time in weeks. She stood at the front door, and I gave her the Sunday paper. We both wore masks, and she wanted a hug. I couldn't give her one and I felt bad. Poor dear. At least they have been on lockdown long enough that they are letting the residents walk in the halls and go onto the patio now. They even had bingo on Friday, and she won some candy.

---

3 May 2020

Mom's dementia is getting worse. She phoned me six times yesterday and didn't remember phoning. She had a nightmare and woke up frightened and didn't know where she was, she lost her apt key, she wanted to know where her checkbook was (Here, and we've discussed this repeatedly), she didn't know what to do with the Census letter she received, and she apologized for saying something bad (which she hadn't done). I feel so bad for her. She constantly laments that she is losing her memory and feels so sad about everything.

At least she can still play her organ, but she doesn't read books anymore. She has several she got as presents for Christmas that she hasn't even touched. She used to read every day, but now can't concentrate. She is forgetting how to use her iPad and can't get into her email or play Candy Crush or her other games. Her world is shrinking more each day, and this quarantine makes it worse. Since I'm still not allowed to visit, I can't help her with it. It breaks my heart that we can't bring her home to visit anymore. I hate this COVID 19!!!

But we are thankful that her facility remains virus free. Tons of other nursing homes are having lots of deaths. Hers started taking temps and limiting visitors early on.

---

17 May 2020

The facility did more testing on Mom and noted that her memory is worse, and she needs more attention and care. She gets lost every time she walks the halls, and they need to help her find her apartment.

They said she's having more crying spells and needs comforting. So, the cost of her care is increasing by $800/month, but they agreed they didn't want to put her in the locked-down memory care unit yet. She can still carry on a conversation, eat, bathe and dress herself, which most of those people can no longer do.

Also, they are now allowing residents to leave the facility for short periods to visit family. We haven't been able to do that for over two months and the administration noted that most residents are overly depressed because family has not been able to visit them. We will have to wear masks, and they will keep checking her temps 2X a day afterwards. But I can bring her to the house for several hours. Hurrah! We are still not allowed in the facility.

---

23 May 2020

I've been able to bring Mom to the house for lunch twice this week, we took a drive out to the lake, and I took her for a checkup with the cardiologist.

She said, "it feels like getting out of prison". Poor dear. The residents still aren't allowed to eat together so she's been eating alone in her room all this time. At least she can walk in the halls and sit on the patio if she wears a mask. All of them really miss the socialization.

14 June 2020

Despite everything going on I had a nice 70th birthday. S came to visit for a few days and Mom was here for my b-day lunch of crab legs, lobster claws, sweet potato fries and cake.

Yesterday the nurse called me and said Mom had left the building and wandered outside by herself. They found her when she was trying to come back inside at a locked door. They didn't write it up as an incident report yet, but if it happens too often, she will have to be moved to the locked unit. Her history of falling so much makes it unsafe for her to leave the building alone.

I've tried to talk to her, but sometimes when she's having those 'spells' she says she wants to 'go out to the street and she doesn't care who picks her up'. I'm afraid she is getting worse every day.

25 June 2020

It turned out Mom has a UTI from a drug-resistant strain of bacteria. The doctor put her on antibiotics and hopefully that will help her malaise and depression. Often the elderly get depressed when they have some type of infection. I've been bringing her home for lunch or we've been taking a car ride several times a week to help her not feel so lonely.

---

6 August 2020

We had a little luncheon for Mom's birthday on Tues. Just A came and we ate out on the patio.
Sandwiches, potato salad, vegs & dip, and cake. And A brought a broccoli and fruit salad.
The temperature was in the 70's and it was really nice outside. Mom enjoyed the socialization and I didn't meet with any resistance when I took her back to her apartment.

7 September 2020

Mom came home for lunch on Saturday. She fell last week and hurt her back, so it's been bothering her a lot. She has gotten very unstable on her feet even with her walker. She is bad about parking her walker in her apartment and trying to walk around without it by holding onto the walls and furniture. When her hand slips, she can't catch herself before she falls. She has a permanent purple bruise on her forehead. (If she was still at home I would probably be accused of elder abuse.) All the residents wear a necklace with a badge to call for help, but she never uses it. Instead, she crawls to the door to call for help!

25 September 2020

We had a little scare last week. After seven plus months one of the workers at Village on the Park tested positive for COVID.

All the residents had to be tested, and we didn't know for several days that Mom was still negative. I had taken her to a doctor appt. and had her here with Ron for lunch. We were worried we were all exposed but so far everything seems fine. She will be tested again later, and they are watching everyone over there for symptoms. They've locked down the facility again until they know everyone stays negative.

I am so grateful that Mom has a best friend there because no one can leave the facility again and she got so lonely last spring. Polly visits with her in her apartment and they walk together and eat together.

Mom lost her key again last week, and we had to make another one. She is losing her memory more every day. I attached the key to a long ribbon and tied it to her walker handle. Now she can keep it in the walker pocket and still use it to unlock her door without untying it. She knows she is getting worse, and it really scares her. I feel so bad for her.

(Mom kept untying the key so I had to chain it to the walker!)

22 November 2020

On Tuesday, 17th, Mom had one of her spells where she passed out and her heart rate dropped to 30. The nurse couldn't wake her or get a B/P so they called an ambulance. By the time I got to Village on the Park they had her in the ambulance with an IV started and she was kind of awake. I spent several hours with her in the ER where they did labs and gave her fluids. They never did find out what caused it but sent her home stable. They don't know if it these spells are caused by her heart condition or her vascular dementia. But she scared the staff half to death.

She was fine, just tired, when I took her home. Thank goodness they have a nurse on duty 24 hrs there. On Wednesday she slept until 10 o'clock and doesn't remember anything about yesterday. She doesn't even remember riding in the ambulance or being in the hospital.

Mom spent most of this week resting in bed after her ordeal on Tuesday but Saturday morning she called and said she felt better. I picked her up for lunch and she complained about being tired still. But the worst part is that this last 'spell' has affected her memory even more.

She asked where Daddy was. We reminded her that he died 13 years ago. She was confused about where she lives and kept asking if we've sold her house and car. Then she asked how her sisters Ruth and Avis were. We reminded her that they died many years ago.

Several times she wanted to know where all her clothes were and when we told her they were in her own apartment she didn't remember she had an apartment. We reminded her that her furniture, clothes and organ were there.

Last night she called and demanded that I come get her. She didn't want to stay 'in this place' and wanted to go home. I explained she was home, that her things were there in her apartment that she had wanted us to get for her and that the nurse had all her medications there. She got mad and said she would call S to come get her to live in Texas. It's impossible to explain anything to her when she has these spells, so she just got mad at me and hung up.

29 November 2020

It is looking like Mom had her spell because she was positive for COVID. When she was routinely checked last Sunday, she was positive on the rapid test. Of course, she had been to our house for lunch the day before because she felt a little better for the first time all week. Ron and I got the rapid test, which was Neg because it hadn't been long enough even though I was with her at the hospital. We got tested again 4 days later and are on lockdown until the test results on Tues.

She had felt awful all week with fatigue and nausea, but so far still being cared for in the facility and doesn't need the hospital. She hasn't developed a cough or SOB. They ended up finding out that one employee and two other patients were positive. I can't believe we were so careful not to infect her and now she may have infected us. Go figure!

15 December 2020

    Mom has completely recovered from COVID-19. She never had to be hospitalized and never had her lungs affected. The facility must have gotten one of the milder strains of the bacteria. She tested positive twice for it. We had two negative Covid tests and never had any symptoms so she didn't infect us.

    She came to the house yesterday for Ron's 65th Birthday. The government started the vaccinations yesterday. First will be First Responders, ie, doctors, nurses, RT, EMT's and any hospital staff working with Covid patients or cleaning rooms. They next group will be Nursing home residents; third wave will be anyone over 65 years old.

    Hopefully enough people will get the vaccine to stop this awful disease. So far we have had 300,000 US citizens die from it.

26 December 2020

K and M quarantined themselves for two weeks so they could come visit for Christmas. It has been so nice to see them both. A came twice this week to visit, and we all had fun opening presents and building a puzzle yesterday. Mom has a bad cold now. She visited and had lunch on Monday but didn't want to come for Christmas. She is very tired and slept most of the day. I'm hoping to get her here today to open her presents and see them before they drive back to Ohio. Her poor immune system is so fragile right now, Mom can hardly walk and uses a walker even with us. She has lost so much weight her clothes hang on her, so I got her fleece-lined leggings and a sweater for Christmas.

20 January 2021

Mom still has a mild cough left from her bout with bronchitis but doing better physically. Mentally she has lost so many of her memories. Sometimes she wants to 'just go home to Maine to be with her parents' and I keep reminding her that they died a long time ago. It is so sad. Then she asks about her siblings, and I have to tell her only G is left. She calmly accepts my answers.

She is allowed to come out with me for short visits although I still can't go into the facility. They have a few more cases of COVID in there. I worry about the state of her apartment. She often gives things away! I bought her a sweet toy cat that is an interactive toy and meows and purrs. Instead of telling me she decided she didn't want it, she gave it away the first day! It cost me $95 dollars. She doesn't even remember who she gave it to.

4 March 2021

Village on the Park is finally open for visitors. You have to make an appointment and wear a mask, but we can visit her in her apartment now. Ron & I went yesterday.

Last night her ugly "evil twin" came out demanding that I bring her some cash and her check book, which she's not supposed to have there. Everything is paid for automatically and they say not to bring anything that is valuable to her. After the 8th call last night, I decided to take her a check book with one check in it that has had the routing and account number cut off. I'm hoping she won't notice because I don't want her to have a good one stolen.

What a pain! After we went and visited for an hour, I called K from Mom's apartment so they could talk. I don't know what triggers these episodes. She hadn't had one for months. Dang it!

She fell on Sunday and has a big bruise on her forehead, so her balance is getting worse, but I can't convince her to wear more stable shoes. I'll probably have to take the slip-on ones away. I'd hidden them, but she found them again.

---

24 July 2021

Yesterday they moved Mom into the "Memory Care" unit at Village on the Park. She is so confused now she couldn't stay in the assisted living side anymore. It was traumatic for her. They also moved her best friend Polly who is now also terribly confused. Polly's daughter was happy to keep them together. They seem as close as sisters. They didn't want to separate the two of them since they are so close. Neither one of them understood the why of it.

Before Polly was moved, Mom heard a man loudly moaning and it scared her. She was crying and shaking and accused me of moving her in with the 'crazy' people. He is the only one who does that.

Several women there can still carry on conversations even if they are confused. I got Mom calmed down and later at dinnertime she saw a woman she knew from assisted living who'd been moved to memory care last month and that helped. But then Mom slipped with her walker and fell and bumped her head, so the nurse called me.

She wasn't hurt and by then Polly had arrived, so she calmed down and visited with her for a while. She was alright when I left last night and was happy to get her hair appointment for a perm today. I hope it doesn't take too long for the two of them to settle in. The young man who moved their belongings set the rooms up exactly as they were in their old apartments, so hopefully that will help. Today when I checked on her the nurse said she was upset at breakfast until Polly came to eat, then she was OK.

I found her at the beauty parlor this morning and she seemed alright.

3 August 2021

Tomorrow is Mom's 92" birthday. Polly is allowed to come to our house with her for cake and ice cream. They are both still confused about why they were moved to memory care, but they seem to be doing better with being there. Aides helped Mom shower and wash her hair, and she didn't fuss about it. She sometimes comes out of her room without Polly and visits with the other patients. She hasn't cussed at me anymore after the first few days when she would call and get mad that I'd moved her there. She would yell then hang up on me when I tried to explain things to her.

We'll see how things go when I have to take them both back to their new apartments, after they visit here.

(They both did fine going home. They had cake and ice cream and loved listening to the player piano. Polly brought her 'dog' and they thought it liked the party.)

26 September 2021

Mom's memory is so bad now she doesn't recognize the facility when we come back from a drive. She asks if I'm sure this is where she lives. She calls after her dinner to tell me that she can't find a way home, so she'll probably have to spend the night there at the hotel. I remind her that she is home. I tell her to look and see if her furniture is there and to see her organ and remind her that she lives there. She calms down and accepts what I tell her.

16 November 2021

Mom continues to go downhill in that more memories are fading. Thankfully her brother, G is coming to visit us over Thanksgiving to see her. I know that will help her feel better and I will take lots of photos to remind her of his visit.

Next week will be super busy as G comes, we have people here for dinner on Thursday, then Ron has a Santa photo shoot all day Saturday. Then I need to get G to the airport on Sunday morning and go to Church where I teach in Primary. Yikes seems too busy. Hope I can hold up.

16 December 2021

We had a lovely Thanksgiving with family. Mom did well and wasn't too bothered by all the activity. Now she's complained of not being able to hear. When I checked her ears, they are jammed with hard wax. I tried drops and it didn't help. Dr. P ordered prescription drops for five days to soften the wax and he will try to wash her ears on Monday. If that doesn't work, I will have to take her to an ear specialist. Good grief, it's always something. (Luckily the doc was able to clear her ears.)

5 January 2022

Mom continues to want to go 'home' to the farmhouse in Maine to live with her parents.

She is confused so easily. But her check-up with the cardiologist was fine. (She had by-pass surgery five years ago.) We got her some new clothes for Christmas, ie. sweaters and warm pants. But it's hard to get her to wear them. She often puts the same outfits back on for several days in a row and they are dirty. Thankfully she gets bathed twice a week, so her clothes at least get changed then.

1 February 2022

We didn't get to go stay with A in her condo at Orange Beach, Alabama as we'd hoped. Mom fell, then got a UTI and wasn't feeling well. I didn't feel comfortable being 12 hours away from her. We did go to Branson with the T's for three days. It's only two hours away and Mom was feeling better by the end of January. (I guess it's good we didn't go to Orange Beach after all. A ended up catching COVID right when we would have been there.)

---

20 April 2022

Mom has been having more crying spells, so the doc increased her medication to twice a day to try and help. It breaks my heart to hear her sobbing. She gets confused and wants to leave VOP to go home to Maine. I take her driving at least twice a week and she loves to see the spring flowers and the cows in the fields. After 45 minutes she says she's ready to go get a nap.

2 June 2022

Mom fell on Saturday and smashed her face. She cut her eyebrow and bumped her right cheek. She also complained of hurting her hip. She was bleeding and they called an ambulance. We spent about three hours in the emergency room at Northwest while they did a CT scan of her head and x-rayed her face and hip. No bleeding in her brain, labs were good and no cracked or broken bones. The doctor ordered morphine for pain and Zofran VI for nausea. They sent her home and the staff at VOP kept a close eye on her. Sunday, she had less swelling in her face but a whooper of a black eye and bruised face. She doesn't remember any of it. Not the ambulance, hospital or falling. It was a blackout to her.

7 August 2022

S came up for a few days to be here for Mom's 93rd birthday. Mom is so confused now that when she comes to my house and it's time to go home, she thinks I'm supposed to drive her to the farmhouse in Maine to live with Mum and Pup. I hate not being able to bring her to the house anymore.

So, we had the party for her at Village on the Park. They had balloons for her, and we took cake, ice cream and party favors. It turned out nice and Mom seemed fine with it. S went home this morning. G is coming to visit at the end of the month. He wanted to see Mom again before she forgets who he is.

---

18 August 2022

The nurse called about Mom this morning. She bumped her head again trying to move the big television stand. She still tries to unplug it and the box that now covers the wall plug made her decide to pull the cord out on the back of television itself. She is positive that it will be hit by lightning at night if she doesn't unplug it! So, they've asked that we remove her TV from the room.

They are trying to keep her out with the others to watch TV and visit as she doesn't use her walker when she is in her room. She parks it and walks around holding on to door frames and cabinets. That's probably how she fell last month.

She also had one of her "evil twin" episodes which the doctor witnessed so they have increased her dosage of Seroquel to 75mg twice a day. She was totally confused, demanding that the nurse call me to take her home to Maine to live in the farmhouse with her parents, and she's also gotten more tired and weak. The nurse suggested that I begin working with Hospice within the next month as Mom becomes weaker. They can come in and help with bathing and other things as needed. Sigh.

---

19 September 2022

Last time I took Mom for a drive she mentioned that Mum (her mother) had come to visit her. I don't know if it was one of her hallucinations, which she's had off and on, or if it was Mum's spirit. I'm glad G visited her before she got this bad.

She has gone downhill drastically in the last month. Hospice oversees her medications even though she is still living at VOP. Her spells and falls have worsened, and she is now on Ativan every 4 hrs during the day. This weekend she hasn't wanted to eat anything and is too weak to walk. They've been using a wheelchair now. I bought her yogurt and strawberry protein drinks and can coax a little down her when I'm there. She falls asleep when I'm reading to her and spends most of her time in a recliner or bed. Her heart is weaker, and she gets dizzy spells.

---

22 September 2022

I spend hours by Mom's bed in her room now. She doesn't eat or drink anything and is in so much pain she is getting Morphine regularly. I read to her even though she seems to be asleep most of the time. I play church music, esp. songs by the children which she seems to like. I spent the last two night here too. But tonight, the Visiting Angels will stay with her so I can go home and sleep. Hospice has sent an aide in to bathe her, and she even clipped Mom's nails.

I frequently wet one of the mouth wipes to moisten her tongue and lips. She is pretty much unresponsive.

---

24 September 2022

Gloria Mercy Spear

4 Aug 1929 - 23 Sep 2022

Mom passed away last night. Her dementia finally won but she was ready to go. She missed Daddy and her parents so much. Hospice was a wonderful help and all the people at Village on the Park loved her. She passed peacefully in her sleep.

Workers keep coming to tell me stories about Mom and crying. I'm spending time comforting them.

We are having a memorial service for her at a later date.

---

16 November 2022

We had a nice memorial service for Mom on the 14th. We held it in the Stone Meadow Clubhouse. K's family, K, A & G came as well as a few friends and neighbors who knew Mom. Ron and I had made a video movie of her life that we showed, and people took turns telling stories about her. I served some snacks and cookies.

We didn't know it, but my friend N recorded us as we talked. It was fun to listen to the recordings and remember the loving things we said. I sent copies of the video and audio recordings to people who couldn't attend.

I hope my experience will help you deal with the future you are facing. Just remember that every person's experience will be different, but you are not alone. Seek for support when you need it, from others and from Heavenly Father.

THE END